The Freshman 15

by

DaMarjay Mayo

The Freshman 15
Copyright 2017 by DaMarjay Mayo

Interior and Cover Design by Katie Brady
Edited and Revised by Briana Chambers, Datosha Mayo

ISBN: 978-1544106939

Printed In The United States of America.

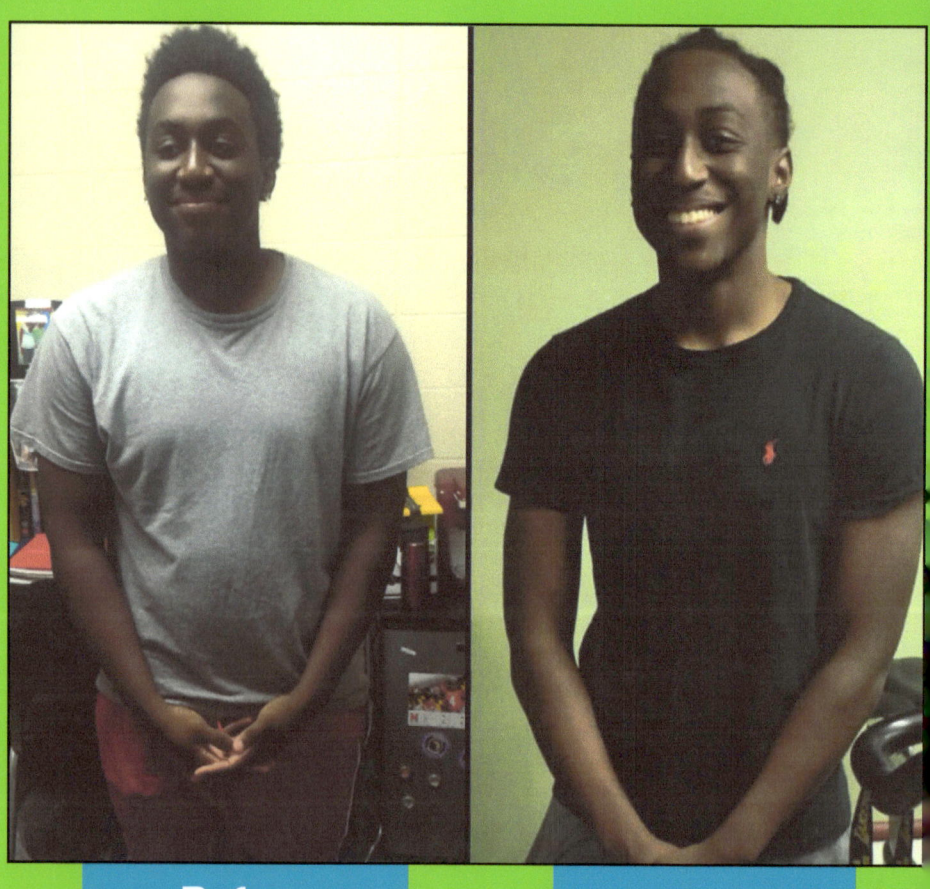

Before
weighing
212 lbs.

After
weighing
165 lbs.

Introduction

Usually, when a student is getting ready for their first year of college, it is an overwhelming but exciting feeling. A step into a new level of maturity, living on your own, developing time management skills, and most importantly striving for a degree. When entering your freshman year of college, there are always family members and relatives that say, "Don't go to school and gain the freshman 15" or you will get the "Wow, you've gained some weight" after

> **...they say, "Don't go to school and gain the freshman 15"**

coming back from Thanksgiving/Christmas break. I was a different story. Standing at 5 feet 9 inches tall, I weighed 212 pounds going into my freshman year of college. As of today, I weigh 165 pounds, and I am continuing to add muscle. I will show you throughout this book how I lost the weight and how you can avoid gaining "The Freshman 15."

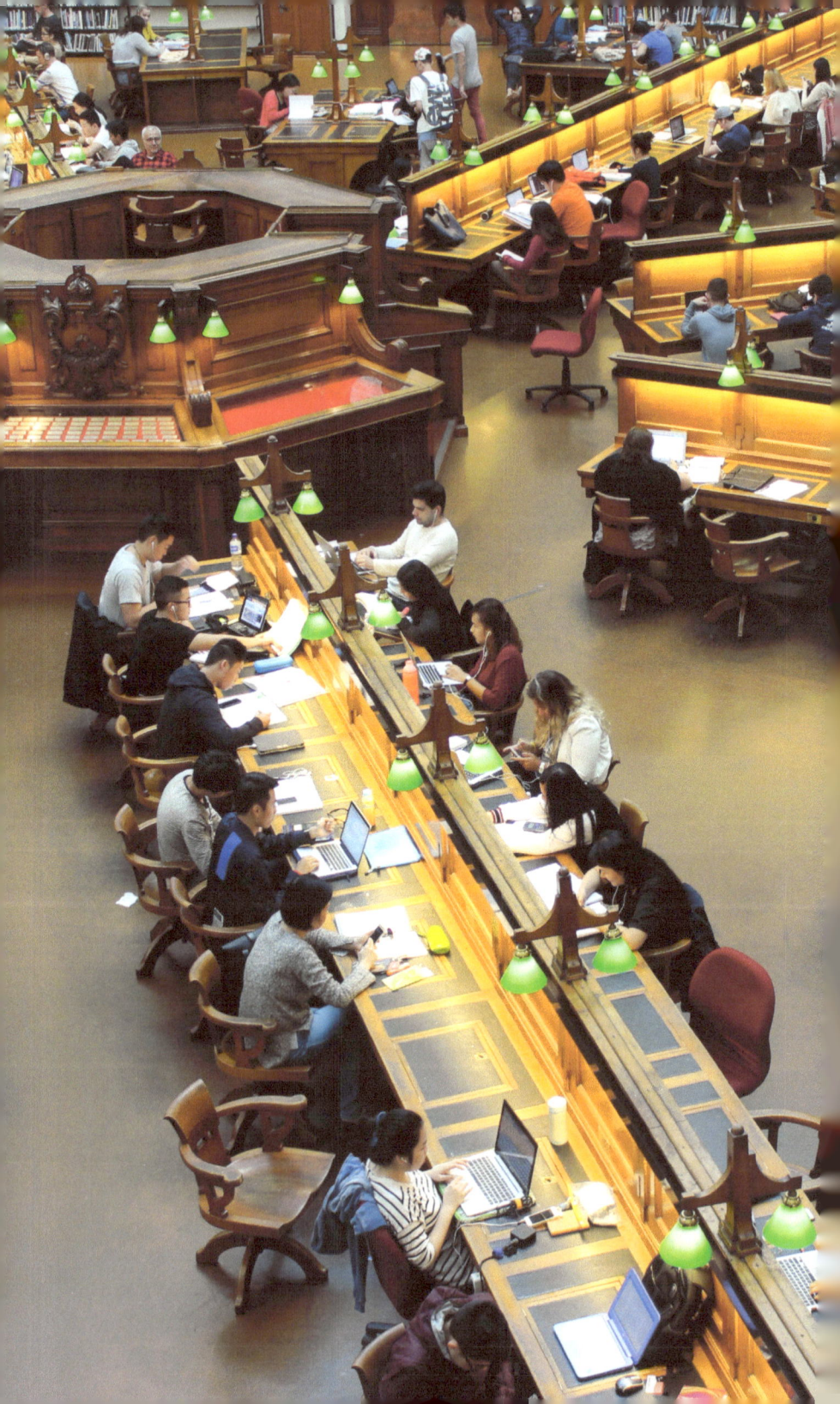

Chapter 1
Preparation

First, as cliché, as it sounds you need to renew your mind. You have to prepare your thoughts and attitude for this journey. If you are certain in your mind that you will succeed and that you WILL lose weight, then you will. It

> **24 hours will be the same 24 hours whether I eat right or eat unhealthy...**

is truly a mind game, you have to have the confidence AND the willpower to do this. You cannot go into this putting in half of your effort. One thing that helped me through the process was consistently telling myself "24 hours will be the same 24 hours whether I eat right and workout or eat unhealthy and don't push myself to get active ". I told myself this because people tend to be stuck on how long it will take to lose the weight and decide not to eat right/ workout because it will take some time. The days will not go by any faster by eating unhealthily, so why wait another day? The next thing you know, 2 months will fly by before you think to yourself, "if I ate healthily and exercised these past two months, I would have lost 25 pounds." In the end, the days do not go by any faster or slower.

The main thing that people have a hard time understanding is that they have to eat healthily while working out. Most ppl think that they can eat whatever they want, workout 30 mins a day and lose weight; that's not how it works. You have to eat right! It is mandatory. You also have to consistently eat well every single day and every single meal with no cheating whatsoever. As I mentioned previously, you have to have the willpower and self-control to eat well every day and not fall to temptation.

> **You have to have willpower and self-control**

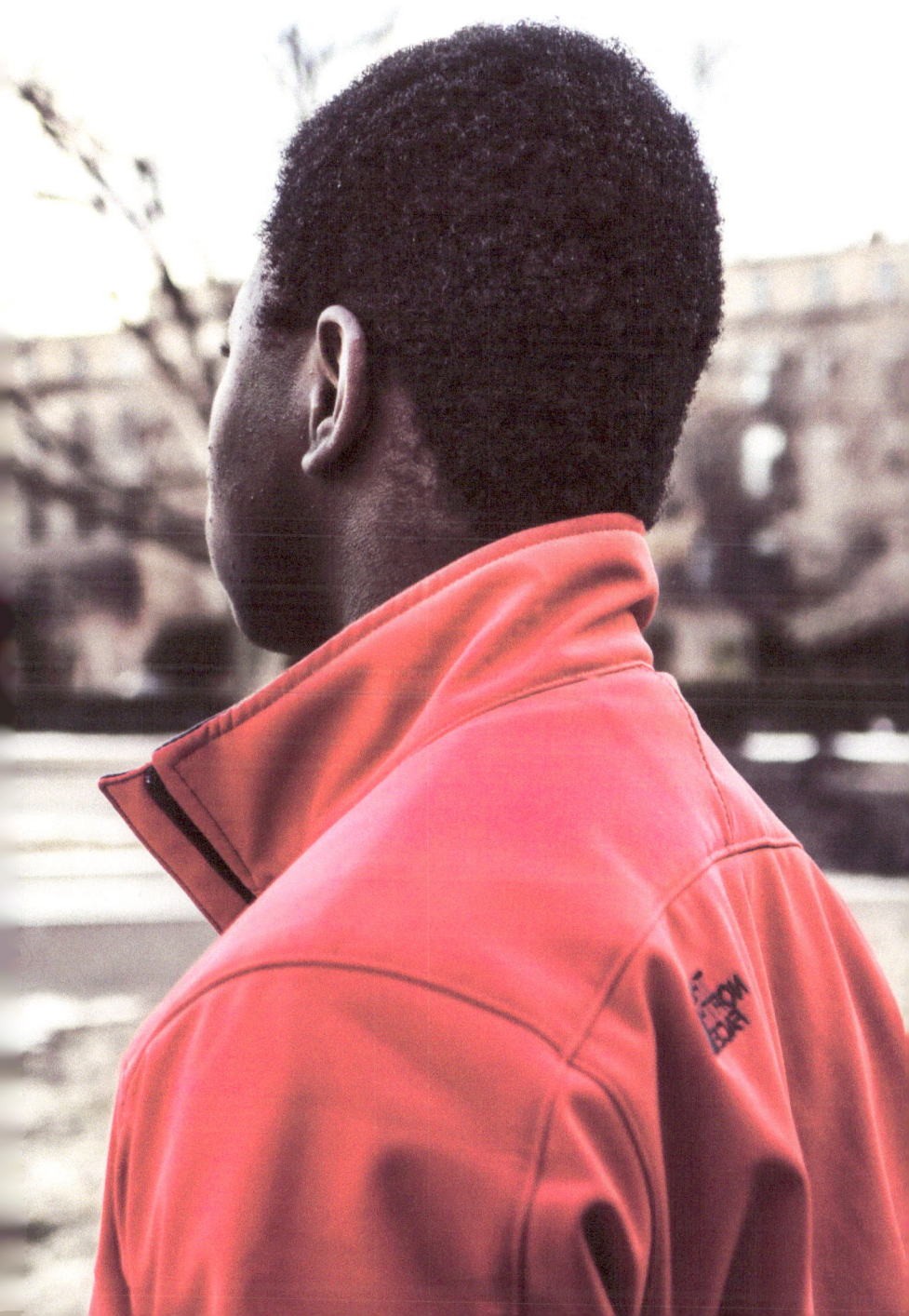

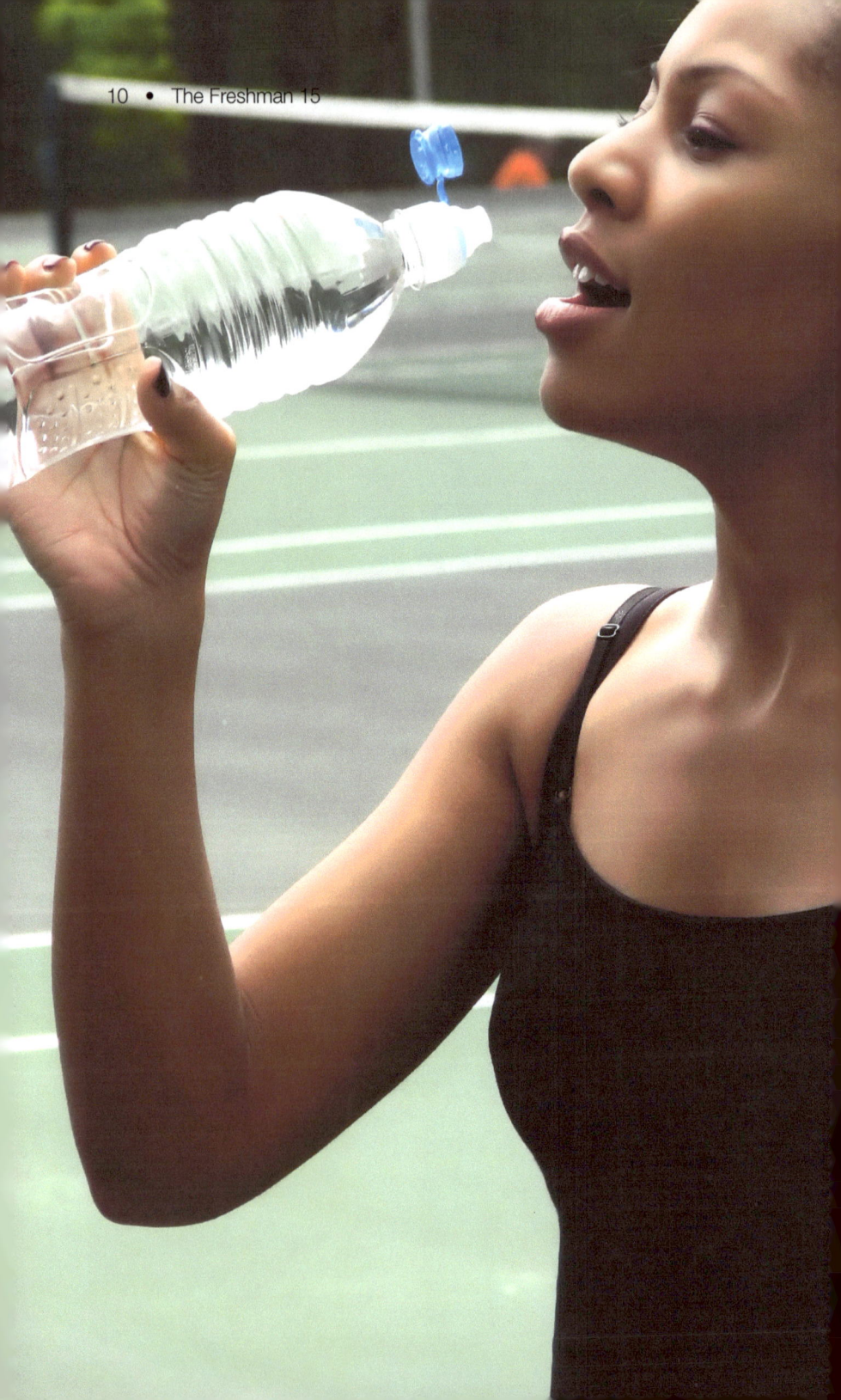

Chapter 2
Just Eat Right!

So now that we have the mental aspect covered let's talk about the eating and drinking issue. For starters, Water is the key to success. You HAVE to drink water and A LOT OF IT. When I first started my weight

Water is the key to success

loss journey, I was extremely addicted to soda and juice. That was one of the main reasons for my weight gain. So I decided to cut those out completely and only occasionally drink Powerade after my workouts for electrolytes.

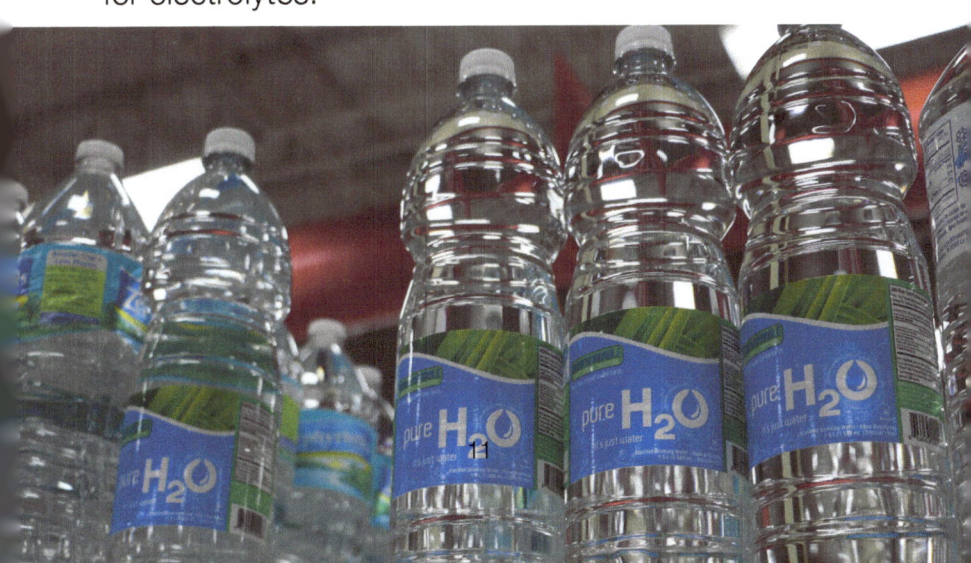

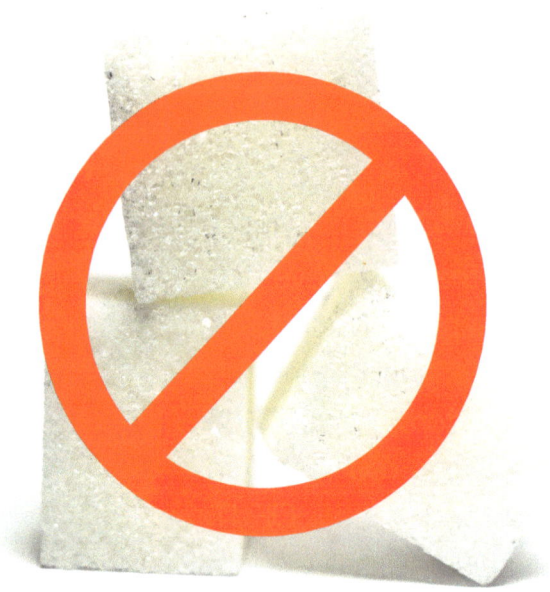

The next thing that has to be cut out is sugar. This is particularly challenging for everyone; sugar is what makes everything taste so good. But when you have a goal, you have to make sacrifices. Sugar, if not burned immediately after consumption, turns straight into fat, and you're trying to get rid of fat.

The next thing that has to be cut down is bread. This does not have to be taken out completely; whole grain wheat bread with 12-15 grains is best. White bread must be cut out completely, this is because of the sugar that is added, its bleached and it has enriched flour. I chose one week during Christmas break of my freshmen year to completely cut out all bread and sugar. I lost 8.5 pounds in 6 days. Some people don't even lose that in a month. It wasn't temporary weight loss or anything; the fact that I was eating healthily and drinking only water caused the fat to melt right off.

Next, let's get into the actual eating, which is the most important part of this journey. I get so many questions about how I ate healthily at school when most of the options are terrible. I always respond with "the options aren't all that terrible and you have to work with what you got."

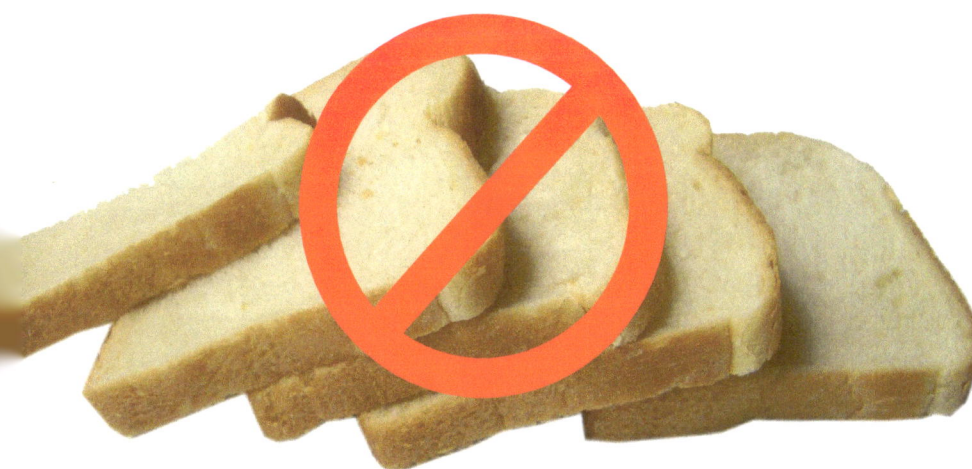

First, you have to completely cut out the fried foods, pizza, burgers, French fries, cake, ice cream, etc. This includes FAST FOOD. You just will not succeed eating these foods; these are the very foods that cause students to gain the Freshman 15-20 pounds. Do not eat these foods AT ALL. It will be hard at first, but after the first two weeks or so, you will get used to it and won't even crave those unhealthy foods.

NO FAST FOOD!

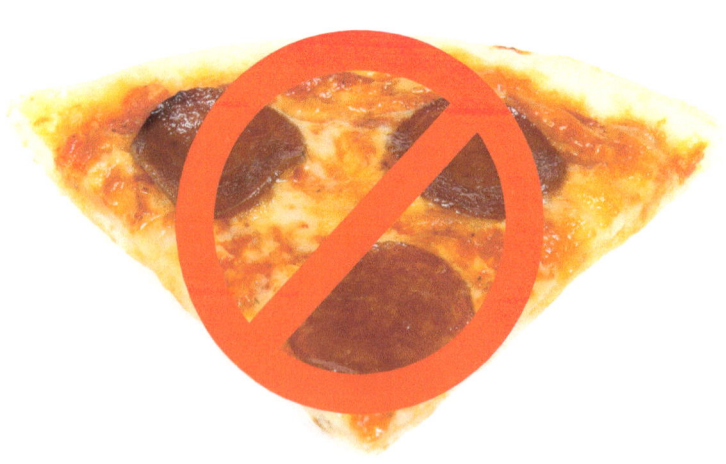

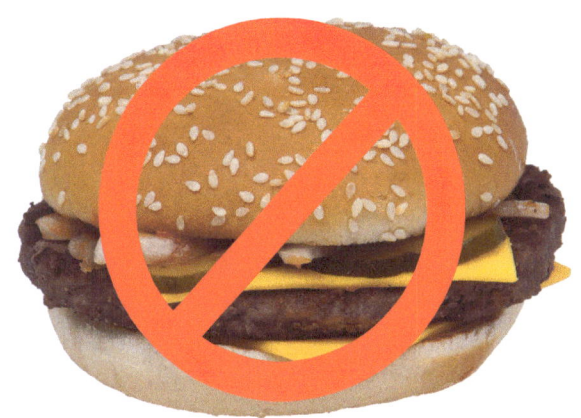

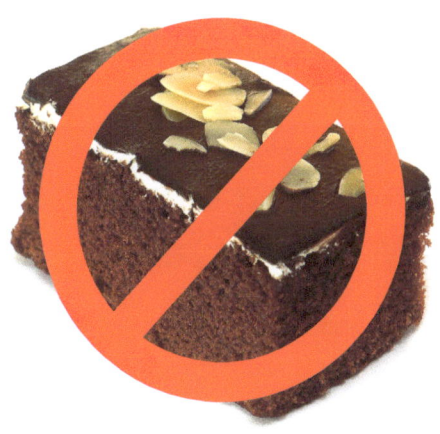

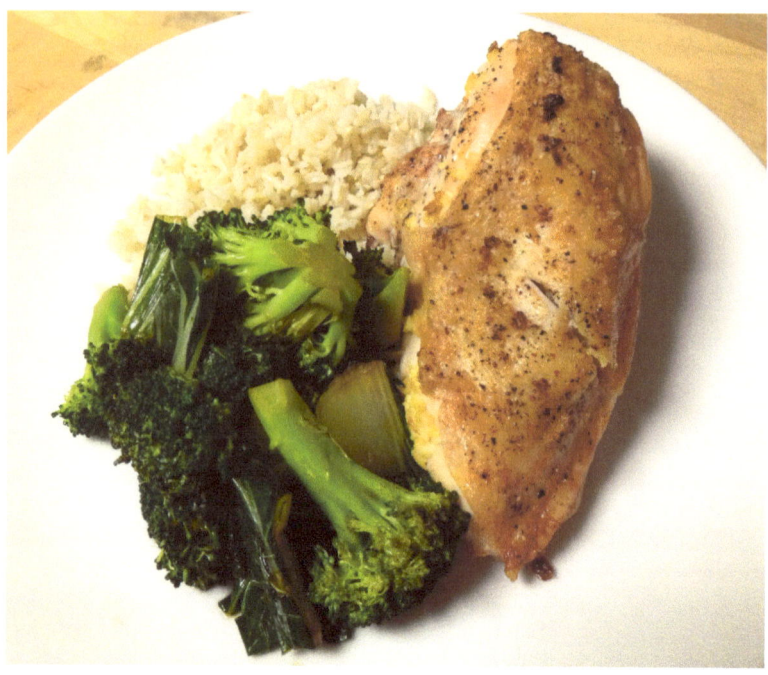

Next, for every single meal, there was some lean meat served. I pretty much ate chicken or fish as my source of protein every single day (baked or grilled

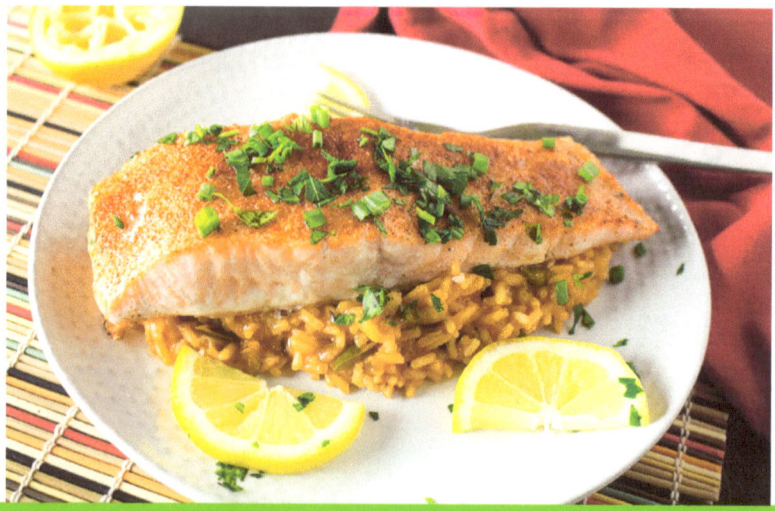

only, NEVER FRIED). There was also a vegetable of some sort, along with rice for carbs. Broccoli was my vegetable of choice. I always added a salad on the side for my greens and only drank water. I only ate one serving of these foods; I never went for seconds. These are foods that my school specifically served; you can apply this to whatever school you go to, at most schools, they offer salad options, grilled chicken, vegetables, greens, etc. It will get boring eating these things every day for lunch and dinner, but you have to work with what is offered, and make a sacrifice for your health.

Cutting down on your portions is another key. This just means eat smaller amounts than you normally

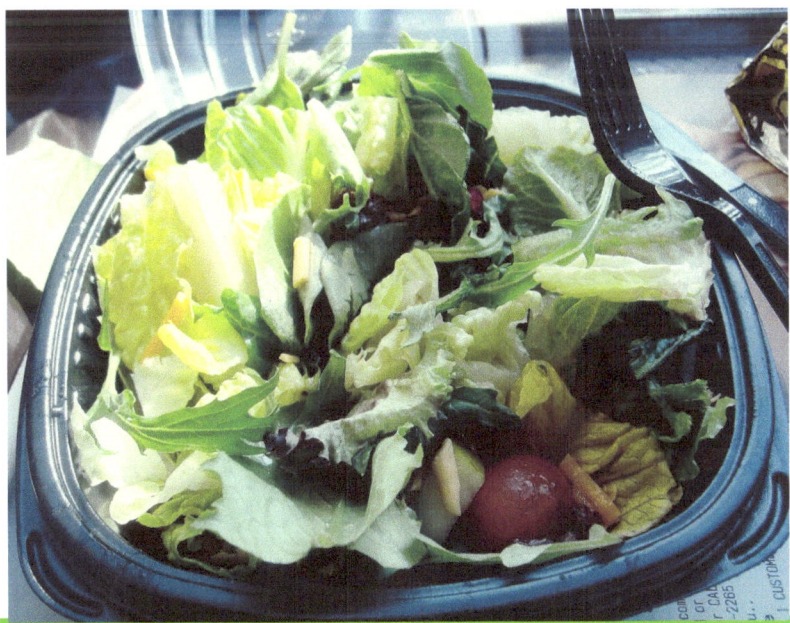

would. In the beginning, you will still feel hungry, but you have to ignore that feeling for the first couple of weeks until your stomach adapts. Now, I am a college student. I understand we go out to eat sometimes and we have fun. When you're in these situations, the same concept still applies. Try to find something on the menu that's baked or grilled. It can be chicken or steak, no bread with some vegetables, and maybe some mashed potatoes as a side or brown rice. Also, most restaurants carry salad. You can never go wrong with a grilled chicken salad for a meal. The

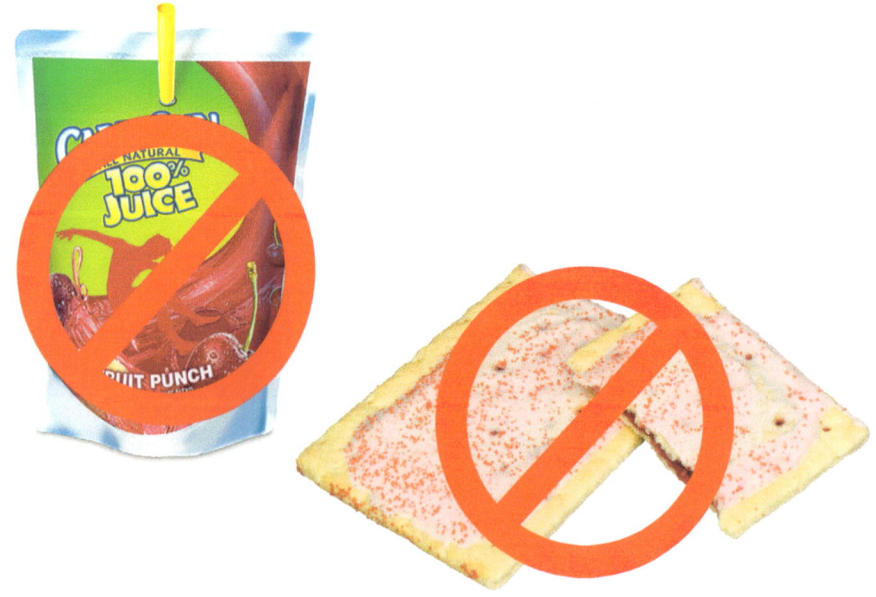

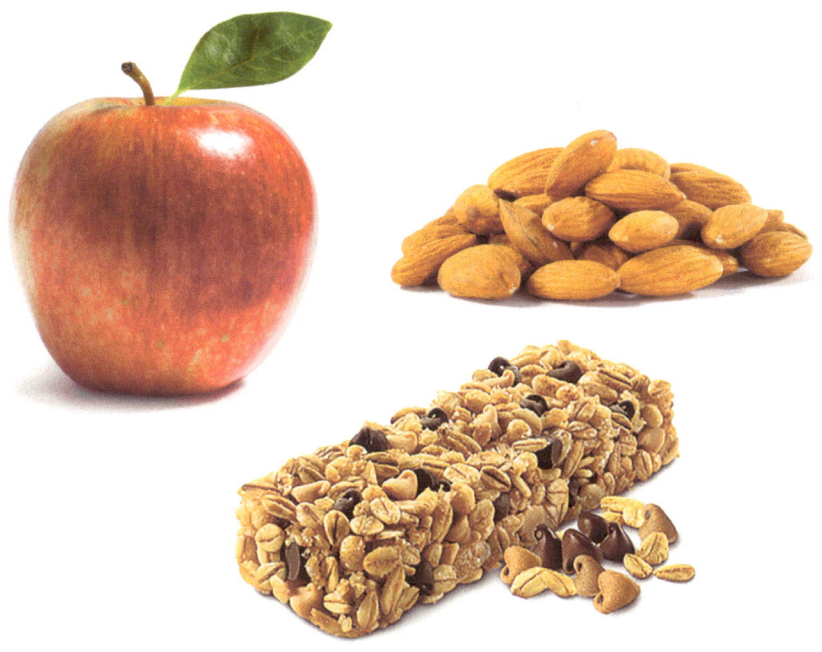

last point I will make is that I understand you might get hungry at night up studying, doing homework, etc., so this is where the strategic planning comes in. Do not let your parents buy you pop tarts, Capri Suns, Cup of noodles, etc. Have healthy snacks ready to eat in moderation so they do not fill you up. Some examples are fruits, Quaker oat bars, Natural Applesauce, Belvita biscuits, almonds, oatmeal, etc. There are a lot of good snack options that aren't extremely high in sugar and calories. Remember, eat these things in moderation not to fill you up.

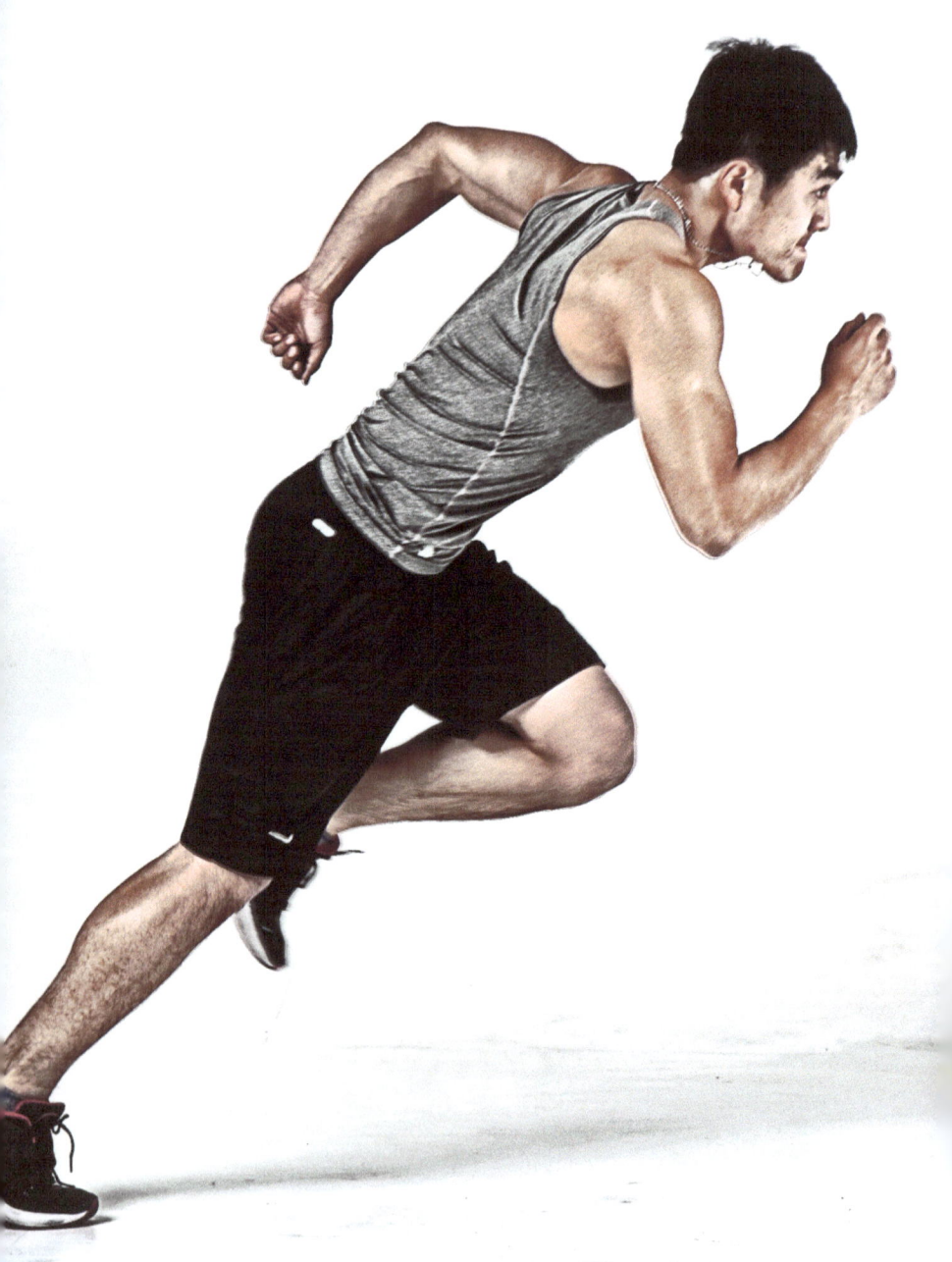

Chapter 3
Get in the Gym

astly, let's talk about the exercise. This tends to be the easy part; the hard part is eating right consistently every single day. Most if not all universities have a gym of some sort. Many people think that this is the most important thing of losing weight, but that is far from the truth. It is essential, but not the biggest factor. Your diet is the main factor of losing weight.

Losing weight is about 70-80% diet and 20-30% exercise. The main exercise that should be done if you're trying to lose weight is cardio. Running, jumping rope, sprints, swimming, anything that gets your heart rate going at a constant rate. If you're a beginner, start

Cardio is the key to losing weight.

with jogging a mile a day, then add in a few aerobic exercises like jumping jacks and burpees, personally,

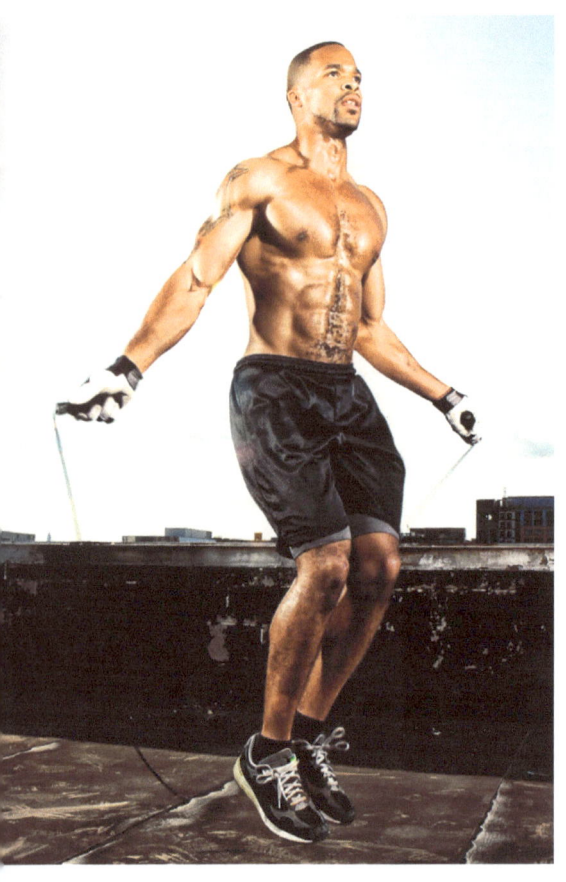

I love to jump rope, and I would run one mile and jump rope 20 minutes each day when I first started losing my weight. The point is you want to get some cardio in at least 30 minutes each day where you break a sweat and get your heart rate up. This does not mean getting on the bike cruising while on your phone, that isn't enough. It's okay to do that maybe as a warm up or cool down but not your main exercise. I see all too often people go to the gym just to cruise on the bike for 20 minutes and sit on social media, you need to be engaged and committing to your workout. Once you are comfortable with cardio, try adding in some weight lifting exercises along with it to help tone your muscles. Make the sacrifice to take 30 minutes to an hour of your day to exercise. Your health is worth 30 minutes of your time. Your happiness is worth 30 minutes of your time. Combine the tips I provided you with the exercising tips, and you will see results. Instead of being the person that gained the freshman 15, you will be the person sharing with everyone how you were able to lose weight, keep it off and become a much healthier you.

Your health is worth 30 minutes a day

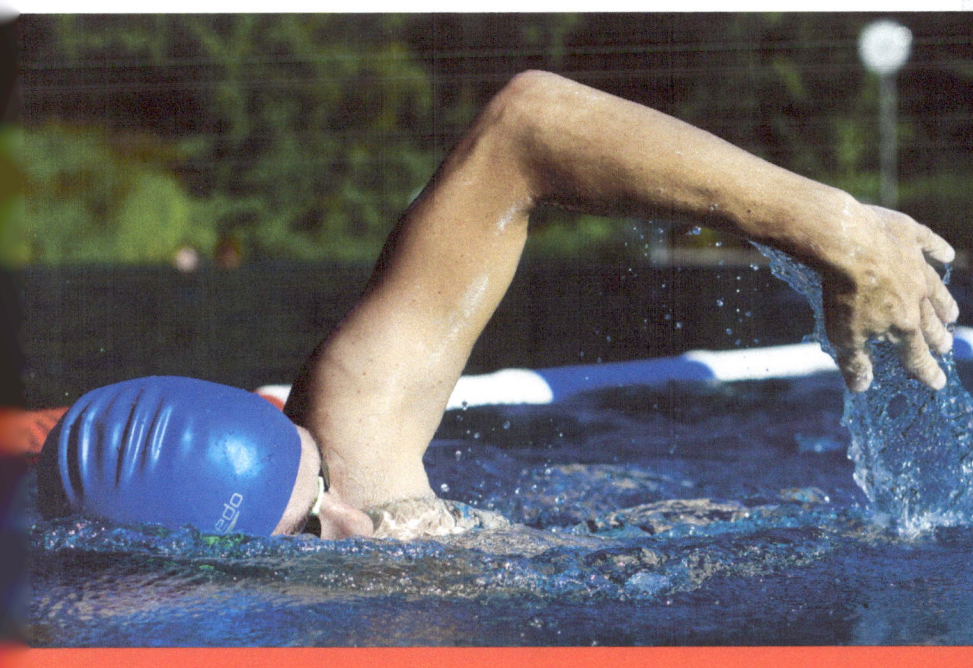

Contact:

If you have any questions or concerns feel free to email me at theFreshman15@yahoo.com.

www.ingramcontent.com/pod-product-compliance
Lightning Source LLC
Chambersburg PA
CBHW050929290526
45792CB00002B/945